YOGA POSES CHART

YOGA POSES CHART HAS 60 COMMON POSES, ORGANIZED INTO THE FOLLOWING SIX CATEGORIES: STANDING, PRONE, SEATED, SUPINE, KNEELING AND OTHER. IT CAN BE USED EITHER AS A CHART OR AS A MINI POSTER.

DIRECTIONS FOR USE:

MINI POSTER ~ IF YOU WANT TO POST THIS CHART ON THE WALL, SIMPLY OPEN THE STAPLE IN THE MIDDLE OF THE BOOKLET, REMOVE THE TWO PAGES AND PIN THEM UP ON THE WALL (ONE FOR EACH SIDE).

CHART ~ LEAVE THE CHART IN THE BOOK AND STAND IT UP AS YOU DO YOUR YOGA PRACTICE OR USE IT AS A REFERENCE TO STUDY FROM OUTSIDE OF YOUR PRACTICE TIME.

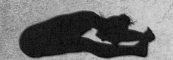

PASCHIMOTTANASANA

Seated Forward Bend

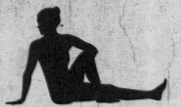

MARICHYASANA III

Marichi's Pose

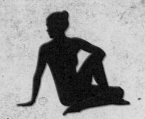

ARDHA MATYENDRASANA

Half Lord of the
Fishes Pose

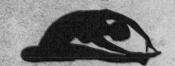

JANU SIRSASANA

Head-To-Knee Pose

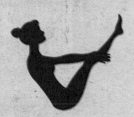

PARIPURNA NAVASANA

Boat Pose

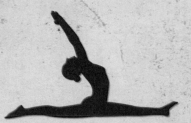

HANUMANASANA

Monkey Pose

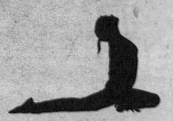

**EKA PADA
RAJAKAPOTASANA**

Pigeon Pose

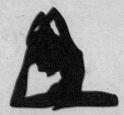

**EKA PADA
RAJAKAPOTASANA**

Pigeon Pose (variation)

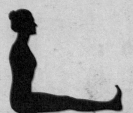

DANDASANA

Staff Pose

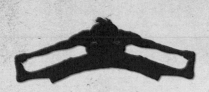

UPAVISTHA KONASANA

Wide-Angle Seated
Forward Bend

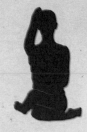

GOMUKHASANA

Cow Face Pose

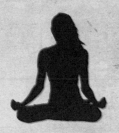

SVASTIKASANA

Cross Pose

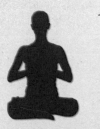

AGNISTAMBHASANA

Fire Log Pose

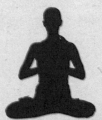

PADMASANA

Lotus Pose

SUKHASANA

Easy Pose

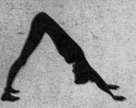

ADHO MUKHA SVANASANA
Downward-Facing Dog

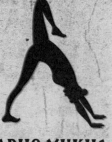

ADHO MUKHA SVANASANA
Downward-Facing Dog (variation)

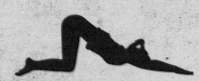

UTTANA SHISHOSANA
Extended Puppy Pose

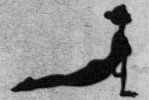

URDHVA MUKHA SVANASANA
Upward-Facing Dog

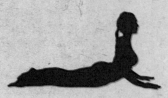

BHUJANGASANA
Cobra Pose

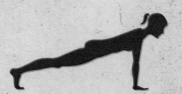

CHATURANGA DANDASANA
Four-Limbed Staff Pose

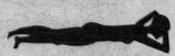

MAKARASANA
Crocodile Pose

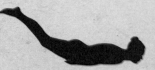

SALABHASANA
Locust Pose

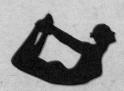

DHANURASANA
Bow Pose

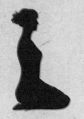

VAJRASANA
Thunderbolt Pose

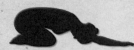

BALASANA
Child's Pose

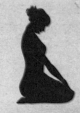

SIMHASANA
Lion Pose

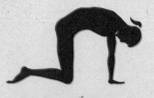

MARJARYASANA
Cat Pose

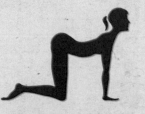

BITILASANA
Cow Pose

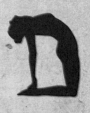

USTRASANA
Camel Pose

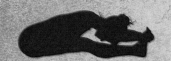

PASCHIMOTTANASANA
Seated Forward Bend

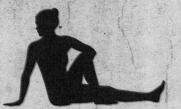

MARICHYASANA III
Marichi's Pose

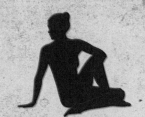

ARDHA MATYENDRASANA
Half Lord of the
Fishes Pose

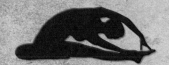

JANU SIRSASANA
Head-To-Knee Pose

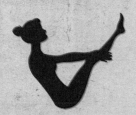

PARIPURNA NAVASANA
Boat Pose

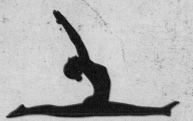

HANUMANASANA
Monkey Pose

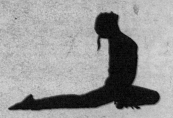

EKA PADA
RAJAKAPOTASANA
Pigeon Pose

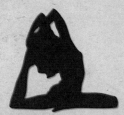

EKA PADA
RAJAKAPOTASANA
Pigeon Pose (variation)

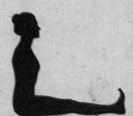

DANDASANA
Staff Pose

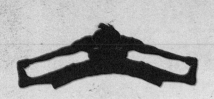

UPAVISTHA KONASANA
Wide-Angle Seated
Forward Bend

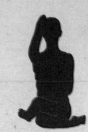

GOMUKHASANA
Cow Face Pose

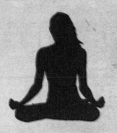

SVASTIKASANA
Cross Pose

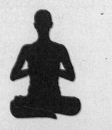

AGNISTAMBHASANA
Fire Log Pose

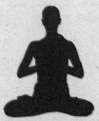

PADMASANA
Lotus Pose

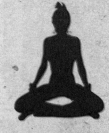

SUKHASANA
Easy Pose

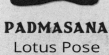

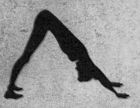

ADHO MUKHA SVANASANA
Downward-Facing Dog

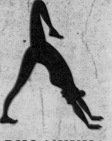

ADHO MUKHA SVANASANA
Downward-Facing Dog (variation)

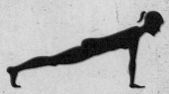

UTTANA SHISHOSANA
Extended Puppy Pose

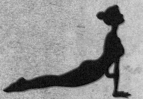

URDHVA MUKHA SVANASANA
Upward-Facing Dog

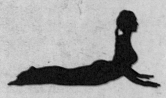

BHUJANGASANA
Cobra Pose

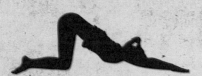

CHATURANGA DANDASANA
Four-Limbed Staff Pose

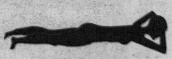

MAKARASANA
Crocodile Pose

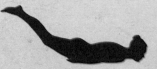

SALABHASANA
Locust Pose

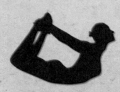

DHANURASANA
Bow Pose

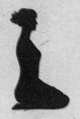

VAJRASANA
Thunderbolt Pose

BALASANA
Child's Pose

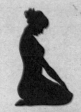

SIMHASANA
Lion Pose

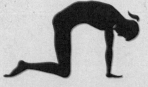

MARJARYASANA
Cat Pose

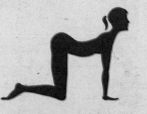

BITILASANA
Cow Pose

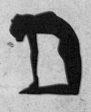

USTRASANA
Camel Pose

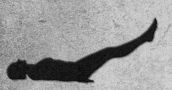

UTTANPADASANA
Raised-Leg Pose

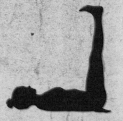

VIPARITA KARANI
Legs-Up-the-
Wall Pose

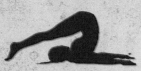

HALASANA
Plow Pose

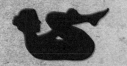

PAVANAMUKTASANA
Wind Liberating
Pose

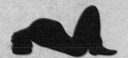

MATSYASANA
Fish Pose

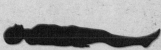

SAVASANA
Corpse Pose

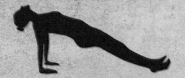

PURVOTTANASANA
Upward Plank Pose

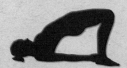

**SETU BANDHA
SARVANGASANA**
Bridge Pose

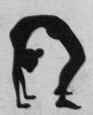

CHAKRASANA
Wheel Pose

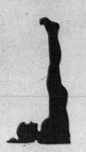

SARVANGASANA
Shoulderstand

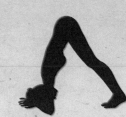

ARDHA SIRSASANA
Half Headstand

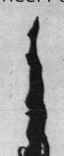

SIRSASANA
Headstand

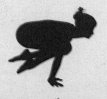

BAKASANA
Crow Pose

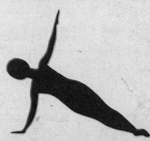

VASISTHASANA
Side Plank Pose

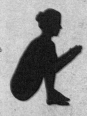

MALASANA
Garland Pose

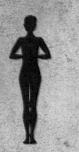

PRANAMASANA
Prayer Pose

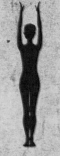

TALASANA
Palm Tree Pose

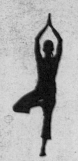

VRKSASANA
Tree Pose

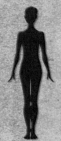

TADASANA
Mountain Pose

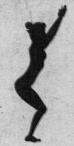

UTKATASANA
Chair Pose

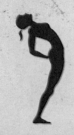

ANUVITTASANA
Standing Backbend Pose

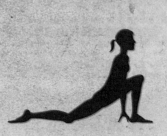

ANJANEYASANA
Low Lunge

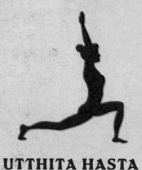

UTTHITA HASTA PADANGUSTASANA
High Lunge
(Crescent Variation)

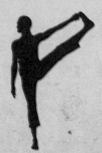

UTTHITA ASHVA SANCHALANASANA
Extended Hand-To-Big-Toe Pose

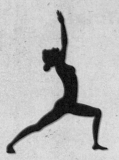

VIRABHADRASANA I
Warrior I Pose

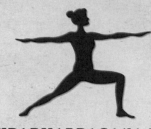

VIRABHADRASANA II
Warrior II Pose

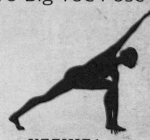

UTTHITA PARSVAKONASANA
Extended Side Angle Pose

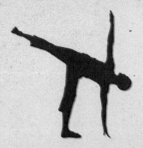

ARDHA CHANDRASANA
Half Moon Pose

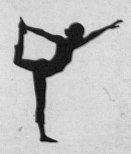

NATARAJASANA
Dancer's Pose

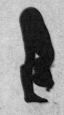

UTTANASANA
Standing Forward Bend

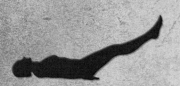

UTTANPADASANA
Raised-Leg Pose

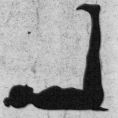

VIPARITA KARANI
Legs-Up-the-
Wall Pose

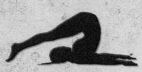

HALASANA
Plow Pose

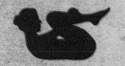

PAVANAMUKTASANA
Wind Liberating
Pose

MATSYASANA
Fish Pose

SAVASANA
Corpse Pose

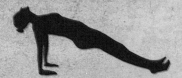

PURVOTTANASANA
Upward Plank Pose

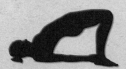

**SETU BANDHA
SARVANGASANA**
Bridge Pose

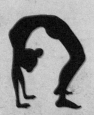

CHAKRASANA
Wheel Pose

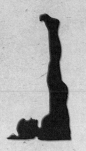

SARVANGASANA
Shoulderstand

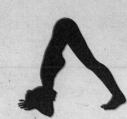

ARDHA SIRSASANA
Half Headstand

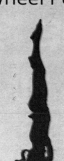

SIRSASANA
Headstand

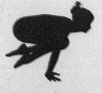

BAKASANA
Crow Pose

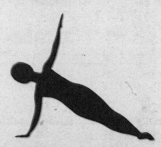

VASISTHASANA
Side Plank Pose

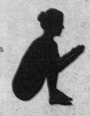

MALASANA
Garland Pose

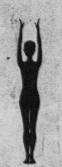

PRANAMASANA
Prayer Pose

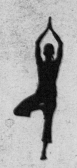

TALASANA
Palm Tree Pose

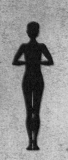

VRKSASANA
Tree Pose

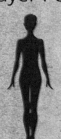

TADASANA
Mountain Pose

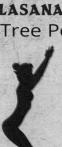

UTKATASANA
Chair Pose

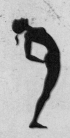

ANUVITTASANA
Standing Backbend Pose

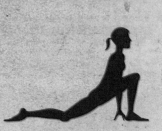

ANJANEYASANA
Low Lunge

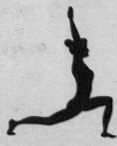

UTTHITA HASTA PADANGUSTASANA
High Lunge
(Crescent Variation)

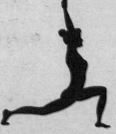

UTTHITA ASHVA SANCHALANASANA
Extended Hand-
To-Big-Toe Pose

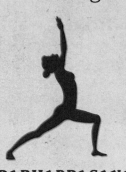

VIRABHADRASANA I
Warrior I Pose

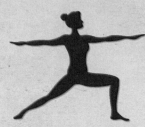

VIRABHADRASANA II
Warrior II Pose

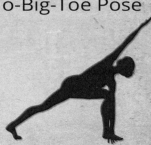

UTTHITA PARSVAKONASANA
Extended Side
Angle Pose

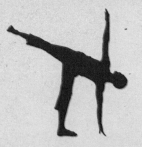

ARDHA CHANDRASANA
Half Moon Pose

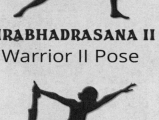

NATARAJASANA
Dancer's Pose

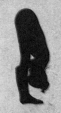

UTTANASANA
Standing Forward Bend

Lightning Source UK Ltd.
Milton Keynes UK
UKRC011010080620
364545UK00018B/55

YOGA POSES CHART CONTAINS PICTURES AND
NAMES OF 60 COMMON YOGA POSES (ALSO KNOWN
AS ASANAS OR POSTURES).

THE POSES ARE ORGANIZED INTO THE FOLLOWING CATEGORIES:
STANDING, SEATED, KNEELING, SUPINE, PRONE AND OTHER.
THE YOGA POSTURES ARE NAMED IN BOTH SANSKRIT AND
ENGLISH FOR MORE THOROUGH LEARNING.

THIS CHART COMES WITH TWO IDENTICAL PAMPHLETS
INSIDE SO YOU CAN EITHER POST THEM UP ON THE
WALL AS A MINI POSTER (ONE FOR EACH SIDE)
OR USE THEM AS A REFERENCE CHART
IN THE BOOK.

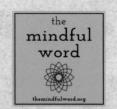

the
mindful
word

themindfulword.org

ISBN 978-1-77380-100-

90000

9 781773 801001